HOW TO KEEP YOUTHFUL SKIN

Susan Su

Copyright © 2023 *Susan Su*

All Rights Reserved

CONTENTS

DISCLAIMER

The author and publisher make no representation or warranties with respect to the accuracy, applicability, fitness, or completeness of the contents of this book; and assumes no responsibility for errors, omissions of the subject matter herein. The author and publisher also do not warrant the performance, effectiveness, or applicability of any sites listed or linked to in this book. All links are for information purposes only and are not warranted for content, accuracy, or any other implied or explicit purpose.

For practical advice books, like anything else in life, there are no guarantees of results made. Readers are cautioned to reply on their own judgment about their individual circumstances to act accordingly.

1. INTRODUCTION

Everyone wants to have good looking and youthful skin at any time of life, either young or ageing. Skin is the first to exhibit the signs of ageing. Fine lines and wrinkles begin to appear, as do sun spots and pigmentation.

Our skin might become dull as a result of factors ranging from sun damage to stress in our modern lifestyles. There's no denying that all of this can hasten the onset of indications of ageing. That is why it is necessary to devote some time and effort to ensure that our skin remains healthy and capable of resisting damage. Many things cause our skin to age. Some things we cannot do anything about; others we can influence. Anyone who already have signs of premature skin aging can benefit from making lifestyle changes; such as by protecting your skin from the sun, you give it a chance to repair some of the damage. Smokers who stop often notice that their skin looks healthier. Easy routines will bring back youthful and smooth skin, such as putting milk on the face every morning and night, putting egg white mask every week for smooth and youthful skin.

The book covers topics from the skin structure, nutrition that the skins needed to daily skin maintenance, to skin yoga, all that take to have a good looking and youthful skin, such as exercise, healthy lifestyle, simple home treatment.

2. WHAT MAKES UP THE SKIN?

The skin is a combination of proteins, fat and water that operates as your first line of defence against heat, light, injury and infection. It regulates body temperature, produces vitamin D, and prevents germs and bacteria from entering your body. The skin itself is comprised of three layers: the epidermis (top layer), dermis (middle layer) and hypodermis (bottom or fatty layer).

The epidermis

Your epidermis is the layer of skin that you're probably most familiar with – it's the outermost layer you can feel and see. The epidermis is made of keratin and other proteins that stick together to form your skin, and it's always making new skin cells to replace the ones you lose every day. This layer also contains melanin, the pigment that gives skin its colour.

The dermis

This middle layer of the skin makes up 90% of your skin's thickness. Known as the dermis, it contains collagen, which strengthens skin cells, and elastin, which keeps skin flexible. It also includes your hair follicles, blood vessels, nerve receptors, and oil and sweat glands.

The hypodermis

Your bottom layer of skin, the hypodermis, is comprised mostly of fat cells and collagen. It helps regulate temperature, protects your organs, and houses connective tissue that binds your skin to muscles and bones.

3. NUTRITIONS THAT THE SKIN NEEDED

The skin need certain nutrition to keep it looking good and young. To help you optimize your nutrition for a glowing complexion, here is a list of skin-loving micronutrients and the best dietary sources of these:

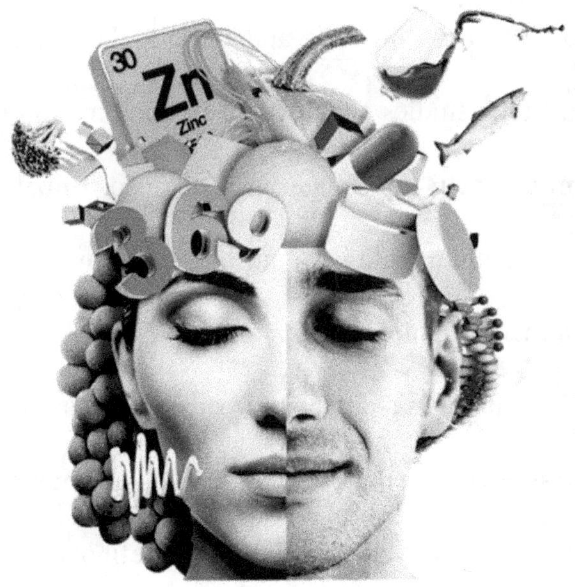

(1) Lactic acid: Another beneficial ingredient is alpha lipoic acid, a potent antioxidant that naturally occurs in the body. Alpha lipoic acid is a wonderful anti-aging mechanism. It has been shown to reduce fine lines, improve skin texture, tighten pores, and give skin a general radiance. Alpha hydroxyl acid is naturally derived from foods (like citric acid from lemons and limes), such as milk. It acts like natural exfoliators to target, dissolve, and remove dead skin cells, revealing healthier, brighter, and more radiant skin beneath. With properties to soothe sunburns, moisturize, hydrate, and calm sensitive skin, lactic acid is a multi-tasking powerhouse that gives milk its skin-perfecting abilities.

(2) Selenium: Selenium has strong antioxidant properties which can minimize oxidative stress on cells and combat the effects of ageing on the skin. Some studies suggest that in combination with vitamin E, selenium can help to manage psoriasis also. Brazil nuts are a great source of selenium, with just four of these providing you with the daily recommended amount of this nutrient.

(3) Vitamin C: vitamin C is a potent antioxidant that can protect cells from oxidative stress and hydrate the skin. Foods rich in vitamin C can also support the immune system, which can benefit overall skin health. Blackberries, blueberries, oranges and broccoli are all great dietary sources of vitamin C.

(4) Vitamin E: vitamin E is a potent antioxidant that can reduce damage from UV rays, support the growth of new skin cells, and potentially reduce inflammation; almonds, avocados and hazelnuts all have high levels of vitamin E.

(5) Zinc: Zinc is a trace mineral, meaning the body only requires small amounts. It can protect against photodamage caused by UV rays and is involved in the normal functioning of the sebaceous glands in the skin. Zinc is found in nuts, seeds, poultry, shellfish and whole grains, many of which feed good gut bugs also!

(6) Omega 3 and Omega 6: Omega 3 and 6 are healthy fats that can maintain and improve your overall skin health. Not only can they protect against UV damage but they can alleviate inflammatory acne also. Omega fatty acids are found in oily fish such as salmon as well as chia seeds and walnuts. These foods also have proven benefits for heart health and potentially even cognition.

(7) Vitamin A: Retinol, a type of vitamin A (and a nonprescription, weaker-strength relative of Retin-A), is considered the most effective over-the-counter treatment to smooth the skin and prevent wrinkles. Retinols cause the skin to gently peel, revealing a silkier, rosier, and more supple layer. Vitamin A actually help reverse a good degree of photo-damage as well as ageing and keep skin looking healthy and functioning optimally, so be sure to replenish what your skin loses every day through topical vitamin A skincare products.

(8) Silica: This mineral can be found in leeks, green beans, and strawberries. A silica deficiency will yield skin that lacks elasticity which lead to wrinkles.

(9) Madecassol (or madecassoside): **It is** an Asian plant extract that helps plump the skin, minimize fine lines, and restore a youthful glow. Madecassol has been used in France for decades to help heal scars and wounds. European studies have also found that it helps diminish wrinkles, restores firmness to the skin, and hydrates skin cells.

Look for skin creams containing retinol. To ensure cell turnover, protect your skin against free radicals, and stimulate collagen growth, apply vitamin C serum under your moisturizer. Use a broad-spectrum sunscreen every day to protect against UVA and UVB rays, which can cause photoaging and skin cancer. For reducing the visible signs of ageing and looking as young as possible for as long as possible, you should use a high effective combination of vitamins A, C, E, antioxidants and peptides that work together to create healthier looking skin that glows with youthful radiance. The most important preventive measure you can take against the sun is to build up your antioxidant levels and maintain adequate levels of vitamins A, C, D, and E. Eating lots of brightly colored organic fruits and vegetables also boosts levels of these vitamins. These powerful vitamins work like natural sunscreen for the body, aiding in the prevention of skin aging and skin cancer.

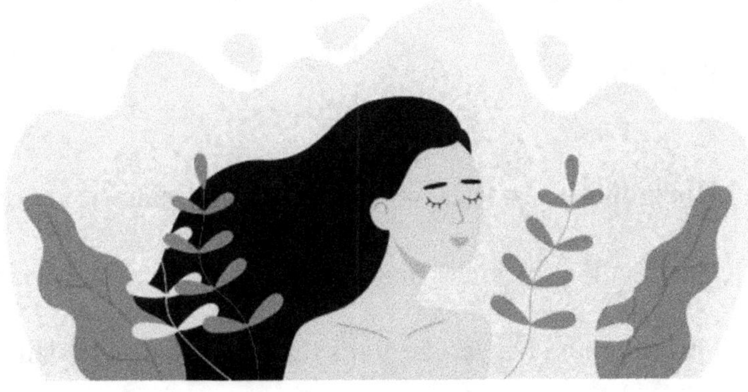

4. THE DIFFERENCE BETWEEN WOMEN'S & MEN'S SKIN

While there are some differences between men's and women's skin, the overall structure and function of the skin are largely the same. However, there are some differences in the ways that men and women care for their skin and the products they use. Here are a few key differences:

Hormones: Testosterone is the primary male sex hormone, and it can affect the thickness and oiliness of men's skin. Men's skin tends to be oilier and has larger pores than women's skin, which can make them more prone to acne.

Facial Hair: Men often have facial hair, which can affect the way that they cleanse and exfoliate their skin. Men may need to use different products and techniques to keep their skin clean and healthy.

Sun Exposure: Men tend to spend more time outdoors and may be more likely to engage in outdoor activities that increase their risk of sun damage. This means that they may need to be more diligent about wearing sunscreen and protecting their skin from UV rays.

Products: Men and women may use different skincare products and have different preferences when it comes to textures, scents, and packaging. Men may prefer products that are fragrance-free and have more of a matte finish, while women may prefer products that have a more luxurious feel or offer more anti-ageing benefits.

In general, the key to healthy skin is to follow a consistent skincare routine that includes cleansing, moisturizing, and protecting your skin from the sun. While there may be some differences in the specific products and techniques that men and women use, the overall principles of good skincare are the same for everyone.

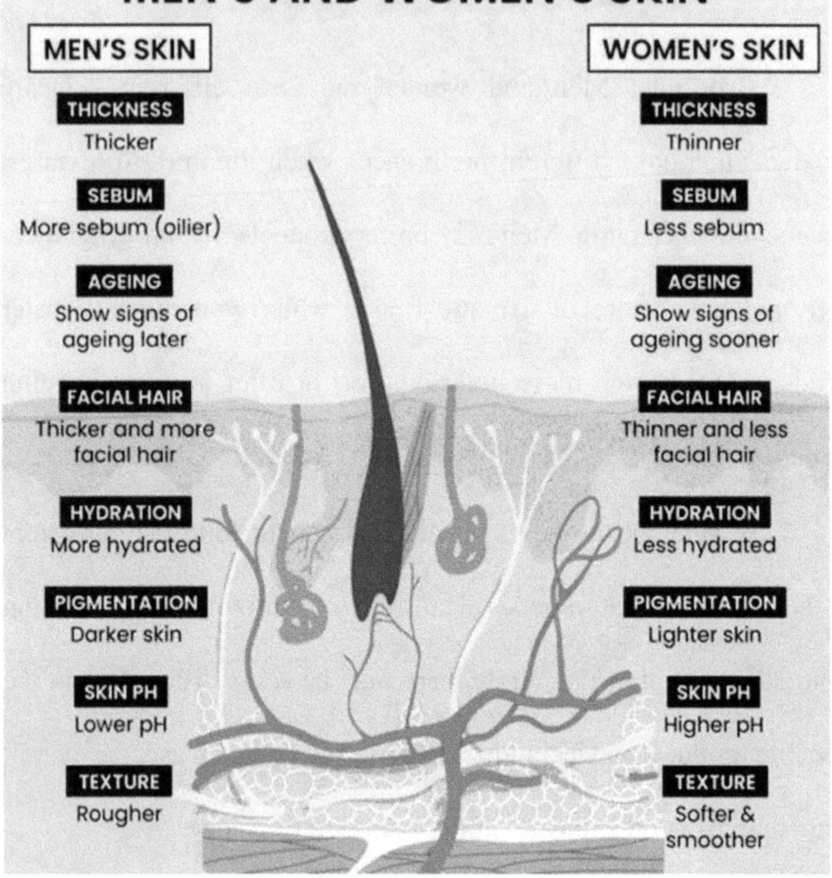
DIFFERENCE BETWEEN
MEN'S AND WOMEN'S SKIN
MEN'S SKIN
WOMEN'S SKIN
THICKNESS
Thicker
THICKNESS
Thinner
SEBUM
More sebum (oilier)
SEBUM
Less sebum
AGEING
Show signs of
ageing later
AGEING
Show signs of
ageing sooner
FACIAL HAIR
Thicker and more
facial hair
FACIAL HAIR
Thinner and less
facial hair
HYDRATION
More hydrated
HYDRATION
Less hydrated
PIGMENTATION
Darker skin
PIGMENTATION
Lighter skin
SKIN PH
Lower pH
SKIN PH
Higher pH
TEXTURE
Rougher
TEXTURE
Softer &
smoother

5. HORMONAL CHANGES & SKIN

There is not a "standard normal" state for your skin, as it will change as you age and pass through different phases. Your skin can change with the outside climate, or with sickness or ailments. Your skin also changes in response to hormones, like estrogen and testosterone. If you have oily-type skin, you may notice an increase in facial oil before and during your period. Acne outbreaks during the premenstrual and menstrual periods are common. Your skin is one of your body's largest and most important organs. It forms a protective physical barrier, regulates your temperature, and provides a route for the elimination of fluids like sweat and oils. Hormonal changes can have a significant impact on the skin, especially during puberty, pregnancy, and menopause. Here are some common hormonal changes and their effects on the skin:

(1) **Puberty**: During puberty, increased levels of androgens (male hormones) can cause the skin to produce more oil, leading to acne breakouts.

(2) **Menstrual Cycle:** Hormonal changes during the menstrual cycle can cause a variety of skin issues, such as acne, dryness, and sensitivity. It's very common for women to experience

acne — especially the week before their period starts. This is because your oestrogen levels are dropping. These outbreaks will usually clear up after your period starts and your oestrogen levels increase.

(3) **Pregnancy:** During pregnancy, increased levels of estrogen can cause the skin to produce more melanin, leading to dark patches on the skin (melasma). Hormonal changes can also cause acne and increased sensitivity.

(4) **Menopause:** During menopause, the body produces less estrogen, which can lead to thinner, drier, and more fragile skin. It can also cause decreased collagen production, which can lead to wrinkles and sagging skin. Your body's ability to sweat changes throughout your cycle as well.

It's important to be aware of these hormonal changes and their effects on the skin so that you can take steps to care for your skin appropriately. This may include adjusting your skincare routine, using gentle and hydrating products, and seeking advice from a dermatologist if necessary. By understanding the impact of hormonal changes on the skin, you can take proactive steps to keep your skin looking and feeling healthy. How to fix skin problems caused by hormonal imbalance?

(1) Prescribed Oral Contraceptive:

Oral contraceptive prescribed by doctors is considered to be an effective treatment for hormonal imbalance among women. It is specifically used for acne treatment because it contains ethinylestradiol which is an estrogen medication. Oral contraceptive targets acne-triggering hormones, especially during ovulation as the hormones work at their peak at that time.

(2) Retinoids

Topical retinoids derived from vitamin A are great for mild acne issues. Many skincare products like creams, gels, and lotions contain retinoids as an acne solution. But retinoids tend to make your skin more prone to sunburn. Therefore, it's important to apply sunscreen whenever you go out in the sun.

(3) Anti-androgen Drugs

Both male and female bodies contain a minimum level of androgen which is mostly known as the male-dominant hormone. Excessive androgen in the female body can increase sebum oil production and leads to an acne breakout. Anti-androgen drugs prescribed by doctors can help you balance out the amount of androgen in your body.

(4) Testosterone Medications

Many testosterone gels and patches are advised by doctors to reduce hormonal imbalances among men. It helps to fight the causes that decrease the level of testosterone in men.

Hormones influence almost every function of your body starting from your physical development to your mood swings. Therefore, keeping your hormonal balance in check will save you not only from unwanted skin problems but also from many severe health issues. Following a healthy lifestyle can help you prevent a hormonal imbalance. Mass-produced, over-the-counter products may not provide you with effective solutions for your particular skin condition. You need a skincare regimen that addresses your individual skin concerns and provides you with products that are made for your skin.

6. STRESS EFFECT ON SKIN

Stress has been defined by the National Cancer Institute as the body's response to physical, mental, or emotional pressure. This stress response may include both conscious and unconscious changes. Stress can also refer to an emotional response. The psychological stress response is composed of negative cognitive and emotional states and occurs when demands imposed by events exceed a person's ability to cope.

A number of potential events or circumstances may produce a stress response, these are known as stressors. Stress may be either acute or chronic and is determined by an individual's perception and response to the stressor, rather than inciting circumstances. In dermatology, stress may affect the skin in a variety of ways, including physiologic changes or increases in behaviours (such as scratching) that ultimately worsen skin disease. In addition, stress may arise from a skin disorder itself, resulting in a self-perpetuating cycle.

Stress has been defined by the National Cancer Institute as the body's response to physical, mental, or emotional pressure. This stress response may include both conscious and unconscious changes. Stress can also refer to an emotional response. The psychological stress response is composed of negative cognitive and emotional states and occurs when demands imposed by events exceed a person's ability to cope.

A number of potential events or circumstances may produce a stress response, these are known as stressors. Stress may be either acute or chronic and is determined by an individual's perception and response to the stressor, rather than inciting circumstances. In dermatology, stress may affect the skin in a variety of ways, including physiologic changes or increases in behaviours (such as scratching) that ultimately worsen skin disease. In addition, stress may arise from a skin disorder itself, resulting in a self-perpetuating cycle.

A number of MBTs have been evaluated for their potential impact on stress and skin disease. This review will describe the potential mechanism of action and evidence for utility in the treatment of skin disease for several Mind Body Medicine (MBM) modalities, including biofeedback, behavioural and cognitive behavioural therapy, meditation, hypnosis, and relaxation therapies.

Physiologic Impact of Stress on the Skin

The skin acts not only as a physical barrier to the external environment, it may outwardly express the manifestations of internal processes. Through its network of mechanical and chemical receptors, nerves, musculature, and vasculature, the skin interacts closely with the Central Nervous System (CNS) to respond to both physical and emotional stimuli. The skin is particularly sensitive to the effects of stress, either as the primary detector or the secondary receiver of the central stress response. The stress response results in the activation of the endocrine, neurologic, and immune systems, with a resulting cascade of events. The 2 main arms of the stress response are the Sympathetic Nervous System (SNS) and the Hypothalamic-Pituitary-Adrenal (HPA) axis. Activation of the SNS results in the release of the catecholamines norepinephrine and epinephrine. This response is also known as the "fight or flight response" and impacts multiple organ systems. At the level of the HPA axis, stress triggers the hypothalamus to produce a corticotropin-releasing hormone (CRH), which induces the release of adrenocorticotropic hormone (ACTH) from the pituitary gland, culminating with the release of cortisol from the adrenal glands.

The release of cortisol, catecholamines, and neuropeptides has multiple systemic and cutaneous effects. In a meta-analysis investigating the relationship between psychological stress and the immune system in human subjects, chronic stressors were associated with the suppression of both cellular and humoral measures. In human subjects, psychological stress was associated with an increased risk of acute respiratory illness following exposure to viruses, with the dose of stress correlated to the risk of infection.

The release of neurohormones, neuropeptides, and neurotransmitters from both arms of the stress response impacts the skin. Catecholamines may directly impact glands, blood vessels, and smooth muscles, while CRH and cortisol have multiple, wide-ranging effects. In addition, the skin is not only a target for mediators; it is also an active participant, specifically via a local HPA axis, peripheral nerves, and skin cells including mast cells, immune cells, and keratinocytes. Taken together, mediators released systemically or locally have been shown to upregulate the production of other mediators, such as histamine and serotonin, increase neurogenic inflammation, increase the activation of sensory innervation, and decrease the itch-sensing threshold in itch-specific receptors. These mediators may ultimately increase skin inflammation, increase itching, impair skin barrier function, impair wound healing, and suppress immunity.

In summary, Stress can have a significant impact on the skin, both directly and indirectly. Here are some ways that stress can affect the skin:

(1) Skin diseases: Acne: skin diseases that are precipitated or exacerbated by psychological stress, such as acne, alopecia areata, atopic dermatitis, psoriasis, rosacea, chronic spontaneous urticaria, and others. Stress can cause the body to produce more cortisol, which can increase oil production and lead to acne breakouts.

(2) Wrinkles: Chronic stress can lead to increased inflammation and oxidative stress, which can accelerate the ageing process and lead to wrinkles and fine lines.

(3) Eczema and Psoriasis: Stress can worsen existing skin conditions, such as eczema and psoriasis, by triggering flare-ups and increasing inflammation.

(4) Delayed Healing: Stress can slow down the body's natural healing processes, which can make it more difficult for the skin to recover from injuries or inflammation.

(5) Unhealthy Habits: When people are stressed, they may engage in unhealthy habits such as smoking, drinking, or

eating unhealthy foods, which can also have negative effects on the skin.

Overall, stress can have a significant impact on the skin, making it important to manage stress levels and take steps to care for the skin appropriately during times of stress. This may include practising stress-reducing activities such as exercise, meditation, or yoga, as well as using gentle and hydrating skincare products and seeking advice from a dermatologist if necessary.

Following are several stress release therapies:

Mind Body Therapies: Mind-body therapies (MBTs) have been defined as therapies that "focus on the interaction between the mind and the body, with the intent to use the mind to influence physical functions and directly affect health". These therapies may ameliorate some of the harmful physiologic changes attributed to stress. They may also help reduce harmful behaviours. In some cases, such as biofeedback, they may result in beneficial physiologic changes. MBTs include meditation, mindfulness-based stress reduction (MBSR), hypnotherapy, biofeedback, guided imagery, and others. The use of MBTs has shown overall benefits for those with skin disorders.

Behavioural Therapy and Cognitive Behavioral Therapy:

Habit reversal (HR) is one type of behavioural therapy, used to help reduce habits such as scratching. HR is described as being easy to learn and "essentially a self-directed approach", although instruction is required. In HR, the main components are awareness (making the patient aware of their own behaviours) and competing response (teaching patients to practice alternate strategies in place of the target behaviour). Other aspects of this therapy include stimulus control, relaxation training, and recruiting social support. Cognitive behavioural therapy (CBT) adds a focus on thought patterns and has shown success in several skin disorders. In CBT, the goal is to alter dysfunctional habits "by interrupting and altering dysfunctional thought patterns (cognitions) or actions (behaviours) that damage the skin or interfere with dermatologic therapy".

7. HOW TO REDUCE SKIN AGEING

As people age, it's natural to experience thinner, drier skin and an increase in wrinkles and other signs of aging. It's no secret that aging is inevitable. It is natural for our face to lose some of its youthful fullness. Many things cause our skin to age. Some things we cannot do anything about; others we can influence.

One thing that we cannot change is the natural aging process. With time, we all get visible lines on our face. We notice our skin becoming thinner and drier. Our genes largely control when these changes occur. The medical term for this type of aging is "intrinsic aging". Other things that we do also can age our skin more quickly than it naturally would. The sun plays a major role in prematurely aging our skin. Even people who already have signs of premature skin aging can benefit from making lifestyle changes. By protecting your skin from the sun, you give it a chance to repair some of the damage. Smokers who stop often notice that their skin looks healthier. Our environment and lifestyle choices can cause our skin to age prematurely. The medical term for this type of aging is "extrinsic aging." We can influence this type of aging that affects our skin. By taking some preventive actions, we can slow the effects that this type of aging has on our skin.

A woman's skin on her chest, hands and arms greatly impacts how old she is perceived to be. In other words, it's not just your face that you need to worry about aging you. To prevent premature skin aging and maintain a youthful appearance, board-certified dermatologists recommend following these simple tips to protect your skin now for a beautiful future.

(1). Protect your skin from the sun every day.

Exposure to the sun's ultraviolet (UV) rays can cause skin damage and accelerate ageing. Damage from the sun's UV light (UVA and UVB rays) is responsible for about 90% of your skin's visible signs of aging. UV rays break down the elastin in your skin, causing a saggy and dull appearance, wrinkles, age spots, uneven skin tone, and more. Whether spending a day at the beach or running errands, sun protection is essential. You can protect your skin by wearing sunscreen, and protective clothing, and avoiding the sun during peak hours, seeking shade, covering up with sun-protective clothing — such as a lightweight and long-sleeved shirt, pants, a wide-brimmed hat, and sunglasses with UV protection. Always

(always, always, always) wear a good quality sunscreen with an SPF rating of at least 30, and make sure that it's a broad spectrum sunscreen — meaning it helps block both UVA and UVB rays. Keep in mind that the sun's rays are out whether it's sunny or not, so be sure that you wear sunscreen every day. And remember to reapply every few hours for maximum protection. You should apply sunscreen every day to all skin that is not covered by clothing. For more effective protection, look for clothing with an ultraviolet protection factor (UPF) label.

(2). **Apply self-tanner rather than get a tan.** Every time you get a tan, you prematurely age your skin. This holds true if you get a tan from the sun, a tanning bed, or other indoor tanning equipment. All emit harmful UV rays that accelerate how quickly your skin ages.

(3). **If you smoke, stop.** Smoking greatly speeds up how quickly skin ages. It causes wrinkles and a dull, sallow complexion.

(4). **Avoid repetitive facial expressions.** When you make a facial expression, you contract the underlying muscles. If you repeatedly contract the same muscles for many years, these lines become permanent. Wearing sunglasses can help reduce lines caused by squinting.

(5). Eat a healthy, well-balanced diet. Findings from a few studies suggest that eating plenty of fresh fruits and vegetables may help prevent damage that leads to premature skin aging. On the other hand, a diet containing lots of sugar or other refined carbohydrates can accelerate aging. A healthy diet that includes plenty of fruits, vegetables, whole grains, and lean proteins can help support healthy skin. The benefits of a diet heavy in fruits and vegetables are many. They provide key nutrients that help support healthy aging and keep your body young, both on the inside and out. Fruits and vegetables also up your intake of phytonutrients, which help your body ward off the damaging effects of free radicals found in the environment. Aim to eat a healthy diet consisting of mostly fruits and vegetables, supplemented with whole grains and healthy, lean proteins.

(6). Drink less alcohol. Alcohol is rough on the skin. It dehydrates the skin, and in time, damages the skin. This can make us look older. While we love a good martini or latte as much as the next person, and both alcohol and caffeine can have health benefits when consumed in moderation, too much can wreak havoc on your skin. Both can dehydrate your body and rob it of key nutrients. What's even worse is that some of these effects can be permanent.

(7). Exercise most days of the week. Findings from a few studies suggest that moderate exercise can improve circulation and boost the immune system. This, in turn, may give the skin a more-youthful appearance. Staying active is helpful in maintaining a healthy weight, but did you know that it has been proven to also help you look younger? Research has shown that vigorous exercise, especially high intensity interval training (HIIT), can slow your aging at a cellular level by nearly 10 years. But the benefits don't stop there — exercise also increases blood flow, moving oxygen and critical nutrients throughout your body, leading to a more youthful appearance. Further, regular exercise is critical to maintaining strength and muscle mass, which also boasts a ton of health benefits and can add years to your lifespan.

(8). Cleanse your skin gently. Scrubbing your skin clean can irritate your skin. Irritating your skin accelerates skin aging. Gentle washing helps to remove pollution, makeup, and other substances without irritating your skin.

(9). Wash your face twice a day and after sweating heavily. Perspiration, especially when wearing a hat or helmet, irritates the skin, so you want to wash your skin as soon as possible after sweating.

(10). Apply a facial moisturizer every morning and night after cleaning. Moisturizer traps water in our skin, giving it a more youthful appearance. And be sure to use a daily moisturizer to increase your skin's elasticity and keep it hydrated. While there are steps that can be taken to help reverse damage to your skin, it is so much easier to help prevent the damage before it begins. Make a good skin care routine your daily habit. Additionally, over-cleansing or using harsh products can strip the skin of its natural oils and cause dryness or irritation. A gentle cleansing routine with a mild cleanser and moisturizer may be more appropriate for some individuals.

(11) Stop using skin care products that sting or burn. When your skin burns or stings, it means your skin is irritated. Irritating your skin can make it look older.

(12) Drink enough water. Water keeps your skin hydrated and youthful looking. Drink 128 once of water daily. Drinking enough water can help keep your skin hydrated and prevent dryness. Another key to younger looking skin is hydration. You should aim for 8 glasses of filtered water each day to keep your skin looking radiant and support optimal health. Dehydration can quickly cause your skin to look dry and dull — emphasizing wrinkles and aging. Drinking enough water each day replenishes your skin's tissue and cells, allowing for younger and healthier looking skin.

(13) Sex active. Having regular healthy sex make your skin glow; keep it looking young and smooth.

(14) Get enough sleep

Another key to maintaining a youthful appearance is to simply get some rest! Getting enough quality sleep is important for overall health and can also help promote healthy skin. When you sleep, your body continuously releases hormones that promote cell turnover and renewal. Use this time to your advantage — this is when you should be using age-defying actives such as retinoids and beta hydroxy acid, which are both powerful exfoliants and wrinkle erasers. But keep in mind that these increase your sensitivity to sunlight, so be extra vigilant with the sunscreen. To take it a step further, consider upgrading to a satin pillowcase. Over time, tossing and turning on a rougher fabric, such as cotton, can contribute to the breakdown of collagen in your skin, leading to wrinkles.

(15) Moisturizing your skin

While water helps your skin stay hydrated from the inside out, you can also help it along by making sure you're using the right kind of moisturizer consistently. Hydrated skin not only looks better, it is also stronger and better able to fight off any irritants. Moisturizers consist of two components to help your skin feel soft and supple: humectants, which draw in water from the air to your skin, and emollients, which help strengthen your skin's lipid barrier and hold in moisture. Creams and moisturizers are not all created equal. It is important to use Clinical Grade products with better absorption and penetration into the skin, also with higher active ingredients, for best results, and backed by clinical studies proven to treat and protect the skin.   These results driven clinical grade skincare products are only sold at Medical Practices like us. When your skin burns or stings, it means your skin is irritated. Irritating your skin can make it look older. Stop use any skin care products that sting or burn.

(16) Stress Management

Stress can contribute to skin problems such as acne and premature ageing. Finding ways to manage stress, such as through exercise, meditation, or therapy, can help promote healthy skin.

8. FOOD AND DRINKS THAT KEEP YOUTHFUL SKIN

A healthy eating routine is important at every stage of life. It can have positive effects that add up over time. It's important to eat a variety of fruits, vegetables, grains, protein foods, and dairy or fortified soy alternatives. When deciding what to eat or drink, choose options that are full of nutrients. Nutrients—like vitamins, minerals, and dietary fiber—nourish our bodies by giving them what they need to be healthy. Visit MyPlate.gov to learn more about what kinds of food and drinks to consume and what kinds to limit so you can have a healthy eating plan. Adults are encouraged to consume some of the following foods and beverages that are rich in nutrients, such as fruits and vegetables; whole grains, like oatmeal, whole-grain bread, and brown rice; seafood, lean meats, poultry, and eggs; beans, peas, unsalted nuts, and seeds; sliced vegetables or baby carrots with hummus; fat-free or low-fat milk and milk products. If you're sensitive to milk and milk products, try substituting nondairy soy, almond, rice, or other drinks with added vitamin D and calcium;

lactose-reduced fat-free or low-fat milk; dark leafy vegetables like collard greens or kale.

Some foods and beverages have many calories, but few of the essential nutrients your body needs. Added sugars and solid fats pack a lot of calories into food and beverages, but provide a limited amount of healthy nutrients. Adults should aim to limit foods and drinks such as: sugar-sweetened drinks and foods; foods with solid fats like butter, margarine, lard, and shortening; white bread, rice, and pasta that are made from refined grains; foods with added salt (sodium); whole milk. For snack, instead of sugary, fatty snacks, try fat-free or low-fat milk or yogurt; fresh or canned fruit, without added sugars. Here are some key nutrients to focus on when following a vegetarian diet for youthfulness:

(1)   **Protein**: Protein is essential for healthy skin, hair, and nails. Eat legumes, nuts, seeds, tofu, and tempeh.

(2)   **Omega-3 Fatty Acids:** Omega-3s are important for reducing inflammation and maintaining healthy skin. Eat chia seeds, flaxseeds, walnuts, and algae-based supplements.

(3)   **Vitamin C:** Vitamin C is a powerful antioxidant that helps protect against skin damage from UV rays and pollution.

Vegetarian sources of vitamin C include citrus fruits, kiwi, berries, and leafy greens.

(4)   Vitamin E: Vitamin E is another antioxidant that helps protect against skin damage and supports healthy hair and nails. Good vegetarian sources of vitamin E include nuts, seeds, and leafy greens.

(5)   Zinc: Zinc is important for healthy skin and hair, and can also help boost the immune system. Good vegetarian sources of zinc include legumes, nuts, seeds, and whole grains.

Some specific foods are especially good for youthful and smooth skin. Following are some of them:

(1) Make salmon a weeknight staple: the fish's high amounts of omega-3 fatty acids help reduce inflammation, which can affect how skin looks. Nutrients like vitamin D and antioxidants can also reduce the risk of skin cancer and help with acne and rosacea.

(2) Hydrate! Don't wait until you feel thirsty: It means you're already somewhat dehydrated. Drink the right amount of water (128 ounce or 8 large glasses a day) make you look years younger, feel better, and drop five pounds without trying.

(3) Go wild for mangoes: Mangoes are loaded with beta-carotene which helps your skin repair itself, stay smooth, and even delay the appearance of wrinkles. When it's not their season, reach for winter squash, sweet potatoes, carrots, cantaloupe, and apricots for the same effects.

(4) Grab those leafy greens: these powerhouse veggies have the carotene compounds lutein and zeaxanthin, which help protect and hydrate skin cells. You can throw them into smoothies, toss them in salads, or snack on these easy kale recipes to get those nutrients.

(5) Load up on Vitamin-C packed fruits and veggies: Vitamin C naturally boosts your body's collagen, which helps keep your skin firm and youthful-looking. Stick with bell peppers and strawberries, among others, to give you that youthful glow.

(6) Low-Glycemic Foods: eating carbohydrates with a low-Glycemic Index (GI) can reduce the severity of acne. The GI index is a scale that measures how quickly foods are converted into glucose. Foods with a high GI rating trigger blood sugar spikes, associated with irritability, tiredness and potentially pimples, such as white bread, crips, pastries and sugary drinks. Instead, opt for porridge, pulses, and beans, all of which gradually release sugar into the blood.

(7) Food nourish the gut: There is research to suggest that intestinal dysbiosis has a part to play in the development of acne and psoriasis. Dysbiosis is where you have either too many harmful bacteria or not enough beneficial microbes in the gut microbiome. The good news is that many foods that support skin health also nourish the gut. For example, whole grains, broccoli and nuts are prebiotics, meaning they feed beneficial bacteria.

(8) Rich Vitamin Food: Vitamin A can help maintain younger-looking skin and reverse a good degree of photo-damage as well as ageing and keep skin looking healthy and functioning optimally. If you're really serious about reducing the visible signs of ageing and looking as young as possible for as long as possible, then you should start with a highly effective combination of vitamins A, C, E, antioxidants and peptides that work together to create healthier looking skin that glows with youthful radiance.

9. PLANT BASED DIET

A vegan diet tends to be higher in antioxidants and other nutrients that have anti-inflammatory properties. These are linked to better health and brighter, more glowing skin. Beta-carotene can also help improve the health of your skin, giving it a healthy, glowing appearance. This nutrient is found in many vegetables and fruits – so you're likely getting lots of beta-carotene if you eat a balanced vegan diet. Some studies suggest that dairy might play a role in acne and acne-related scarring. By eliminating dairy from your diet, you might see increased healing of acne and scars.

Something labelled as vegan does not at all imply it is healthy. Pasta and sauce, and peanut butter and jelly- are vegan meal options, however not health-promoting. A vegan diet may be higher in carbohydrates, gluten, sugar, and pro-inflammatory omega-6 fatty acids. What are the health risks of being vegan?

The one thing to take into consideration is that, if you aren't consuming any meat or dairy products, you won't be able to take advantage of the skin-improving benefits of collagen as easily. Collagen is a protein that naturally gives our skin volume – it is the most abundant protein in the human body. As we get older, our collagen levels rapidly decline, which makes our skin appear saggy and develop wrinkles. You can take a collagen supplement to help fight wrinkles- however, many of these supplements aren't vegan-friendly, since they're also derived from the connective tissues of animals. There are numerous plant-based collagen supplements out there to take advantage of if you are a vegan. Plus, if you're eating a vegan diet, you probably are consuming more vitamin C, lysine, antioxidants, and other plant-based nutrients that can help improve your body's natural production of collagen without having to consume any extra.

The other problem is that it is hard to keep up with vital health-restorative anti-inflammatory nutrients with a vegan diet. The community of health-seekers is dealing with higher levels of inflammation in their bodies, and the vegan diet is largely absent or low in key nutrients that quench inflammation: omega-3 fatty acids. There are plant/algae sources of omega-three fatty acids; however, in a state of disease, the need for high-dose fish oil to quench an inflammatory process may be very great indeed.

Another disadvantage of a vegan diet is it is relatively low in energy-promoting mitochondrial nutrients such as B12, carnitine, coq10, and zinc, to name a few. Dysfunction in your mitochondria contributes to many chronic diseases, and it has been implicated in at least one theory of ageing. Eating a diet low in mitochondrial nutrients may be one that further promotes mitochondrial dysfunction or simply does not afford the ingredients for mitochondrial healing and restoration so often needed for deep healing. Some mitochondrial powerhouse foods such as salmon and liver/organ meats are not vegan. If you consider being a vegan, it will likely also require careful supplementation with mitochondria-promoting nutrients and omega-3 fatty acids.

The biggest health risk of going vegan has to do with muscle loss as a result of inadequate protein intake. Eating meat is often considered the best way to consume large amounts of protein, but as long as you pay attention to what you're consuming, you can get all the protein you need as a vegan. A well-balanced plant-based diet should include proteins like pulses, seeds, nuts, beans, and quinoa. All of these offer plenty of protein. It's important to note that it's not just consuming large amounts of protein that help prevent or reverse muscle loss, either. Muscle loss with ageing typically occurs in people who have a high-calorie intake from processed foods as well as from a sedentary lifestyle. By making healthy diet choices and keeping up with your exercise routine, you shouldn't notice any difference in your muscle loss from that of a person who consumes meat.

Vitamin B12 deficiency is another major concern. B12 only comes from animal-based foods and, according to Harvard University, is essential for maintaining our nervous system, DNA, red blood cell formation, glucose metabolism, regulating new cell growth, and aiding in our cognition. Without adequate amounts of B12, you can suffer some pretty serious health consequences. You can combat this by consuming foods fortified with B12 (such as breakfast cereals, certain plant milk, and some soy products). You can take a plant-based B12 supplement, too.

Calcium is another nutrient in which vegans tend to be deficient. It is essential for blood, bone, heart, dental, and nerve health. The most obvious source of calcium is dairy, but you can also get all the calcium you need from things like green, leafy vegetables (broccoli and cabbage are two of the best – spinach also has lots of calcium but the body has a harder time digesting it), calcium-set tofu, kale, and sesame seeds. Oranges and figs are high in calcium as well.

You will also need to make sure you are taking extra steps to get the essential fatty acids your body needs. Vegans are often deficient in the essential omega-3 fatty acids, particularly the DHA and EPA subtypes. These are most notably found in fish, but you can consume them in a vegan-only diet by consuming products like spirulina and chlorella.

Vitamin D is another nutrient to pay attention to. You can take it as a supplement (but make sure it's vegan-friendly). Cereals tend to be fortified with vitamin D but one of the best ways to get the vitamin D you need is to spend lots of time outdoors, in the sun.

Some vegans turn to soy or plant-based meats as a substitute for meat products in their diet. These are fine but check the ingredients list. While soy can be a good substitute in moderation, you'll want to avoid it if you have any acne issues. Soy can lead to hormonal imbalances that can result in unpleasant breakouts.

10. EXERCISE FOR BETTER SKIN

Exercise not only appears to keep skin younger, but it may also even reverse skin ageing. To promote youthful skin through exercise, aim for at least 30 minutes of moderate-intensity exercise most days of the week. This can include activities such as jogging, cycling, swimming, or dancing. While exercise alone cannot completely reverse the signs of ageing, regular physical activity can improve the health and appearance of your skin. Here are some ways that exercise can benefit your skin:

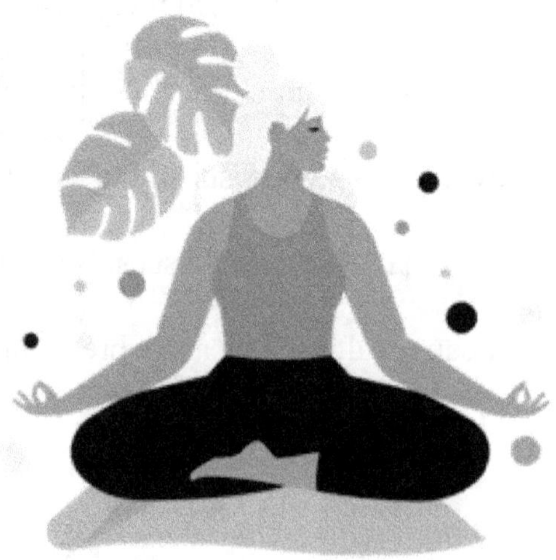

(1) ***Increased Blood Flow:*** Exercise increases blood flow to the skin, which helps deliver oxygen and nutrients to skin cells. This can improve skin health and give it a youthful glow.

(2) ***Reduced Stress:*** Stress cause premature ageing and skin damage. Exercise reduces stress levels; improve overall skin health.

(3) ***Improved Circulation:*** Regular exercise improve circulation, which can help flush out toxins and waste products from skin cells, leading to clearer and brighter skin.

(4) ***Increased Collagen Production:*** Collagen is a protein that gives skin its elasticity and firmness. Regular exercise can increase collagen production, which improves skin elasticity and reduce the appearance of fine lines and wrinkles.

(5) ***Reduced Inflammation:*** Chronic inflammation contribute to skin damage and ageing. Exercise can help reduce inflammation throughout the body, including in the skin.

Our skin changes as the years advance, resulting in wrinkles, crow's feet and sagging. This occurs because of changes within our layers of skin. After about age 40, most of us begin to experience a thickening of our stratum corneum, the final, protective, outer layer of the epidermis, itself the top layer of our skin. The stratum corneum is the portion of the skin that you see and feel. Composed mostly of dead skin cells and some collagen, it gets drier, flakier and denser with age. At the same time, the layer of skin beneath the epidermis, the dermis, begins to thin. It loses cells and elasticity, giving the skin a more translucent and often saggier appearance. These changes are independent of any skin damage from the sun. They are solely the result of the passage of time. Recently, researchers at McMaster University in Ontario found that after age 40, the men and women who exercised frequently had markedly thinner, healthier stratum corneum and thicker dermis layers in their skin. Their skin was much closer in composition to that of the 20- and 30-year-olds than to that of others of their age, even if they were past age 65. Exercise could reverse aging for a much younger person and skin. Working muscles will generate certain substances, such as myokines. These substance enter the bloodstream and jump-start changes in cells far from the muscles additional. Myokines and substances are also involved in the skin changes related to exercise.

P A G E | **49**

11. FACIAL YOGA EXERCISES

Since the skin is the body's greatest organ, it necessitates more than just product application. While the latter is a simple but important approach to good skin, it takes a deeper, more holistic approach to ensure that the nutrients in your skincare are effectively disseminated throughout all layers of the skin, allowing your inner beauty to come through. Eating fresh and seasonal foods, exercising, and having a healthy, balanced lifestyle is all a part of this. Facial Yoga, a mindful practice that allows you to treat your skin with kindness while reconnecting with your inner self, is one way to do so. Facial yoga can be extremely beneficial for those who want glowing, youthful skin; and you may do these exercises anywhere and at any time. It helps a person tone and isolate facial muscles and gives us those perfect expressions. Here are 5 face yoga exercises to help you get youthful skin:

(1) Puff Your Cheeks:

Inhale through your mouth, stretching your breath from cheek to cheek, and then exhale. These simple actions will help strengthen the cheek muscles and keep them from looking hollow. Regularly perform this exercise to achieve lifted and plumped cheeks.

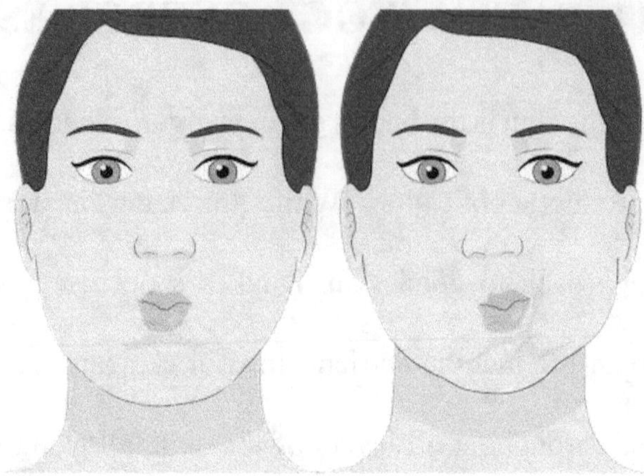

(2) Smile:

Extend your lips as far as possible, as if you're going to kiss, and then grin broadly. Every day, do at least 15 repetitions. This workout targets your cheeks and chin at the same time. When these muscles are used frequently and in a precise way, they can help you achieve a youthful jawline and flushed cheeks.

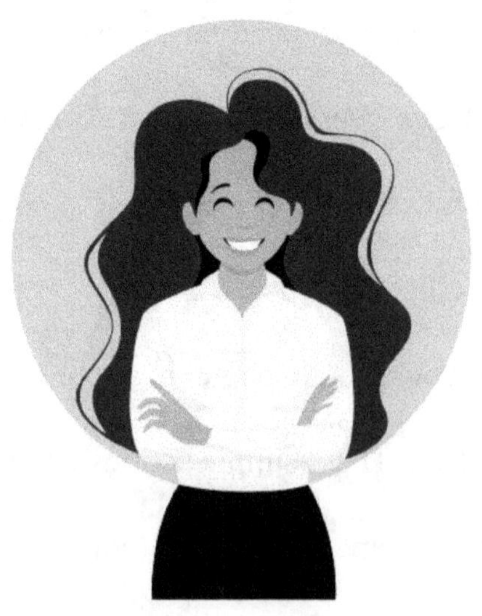

SUSAN SU © 2023

(3) Lift Your Eyebrows:

Place each hand's index finger half an inch above the brows. Lift your brows upwards while pressing them downwards with your fingertips. Repeat this ten to twelve times per day. Because our forehead is the first location where wrinkles occur, completing this specific exercise will tone those muscles, relax tension, and lessen the appearance of wrinkles.

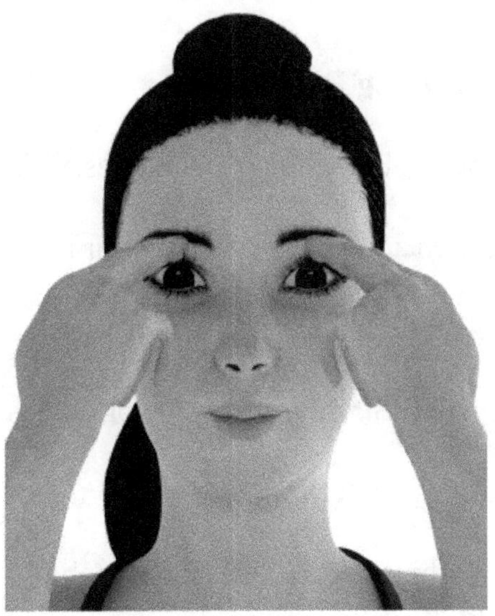

(4) Stretching The Eyelids:

Raise your brows and look upwards at the same moment. Then, while still looking up, softly close your eyelids. This stretching exercise can help keep our eyelids tight as we get older because they tend to droop.

SUSAN SU © 2023

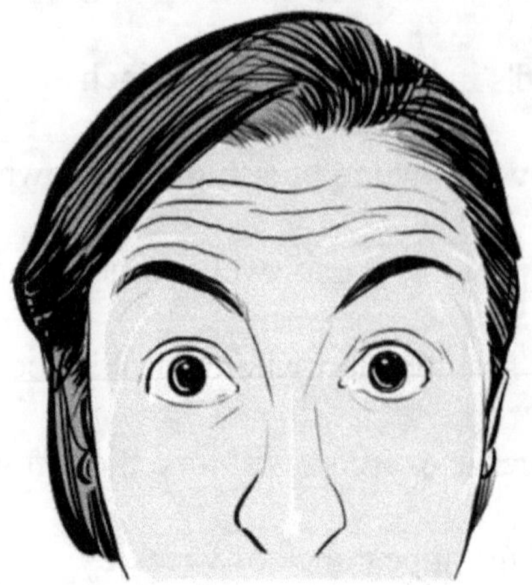

(5) Yogic Breathing Exercise:

Without yogic breathing techniques, facial yoga is inadequate. The skin and body, as well as our moods, are affected by respiratory changes. For example, shallow breathing makes the skin appear paler. Stress in today's world constantly disturbs the natural breathing pattern, diminishing Prana, the life-giving energy. Deep breathing techniques, such as abdominal breathing and alternative nostril breathing, can help restore this equilibrium.

12. MILK TREATMENT FOR YOUTHFUL SKIN

When it comes to skincare, Korea is the land of milk and honey—and we mean that quite literally. It's no secret that raw ingredients like milk, honey, fruits, vegetables, oils, and other natural products are used for their skin-enhancing perks in nearly every Korean skincare brand. Try this celebrity-inspired milk skincare method for milky-smooth, radiant skin. If your goal this year is brighter, smoother, lit-from-within skin, then pour yourself a glass of milk. Cleansing your face every night with milk for a pearly, porcelain complexion. Moisturizing, exfoliating, and lightening, the benefits of milk for skin are tried and true. After all, legend has it that milk baths were the secret to Cleopatra's timelessly youthful, radiant, and wrinkle-free skin.

The first source of nutrition for both humans and animals, milk is unsurprisingly chock full of health and beauty perks. Vitamins A and B6, potassium, and biotin help moisturize dry skin and promote new healthy cells; vitamin D, magnesium, selenium (which has antioxidant properties), and lactic acid all work together to keep skin youthful, strengthen elasticity, diminish fine lines, and exfoliate dead skin. For the acne-prone, milk helps gently exfoliate and treat breakouts; on the other end of the spectrum, it draws out sebum and de-gunks clogged pores in oily skin. Of all these nutrients, we're paying special attention to lactic acid, a popular ingredient in many skincare products. Lactic acid is an alpha hydroxy acid, and don't worry, it's safe for your skin. Naturally derived from foods (like citric acid from lemons and limes), AHAs act like natural exfoliators to target, dissolve, and remove dead skin cells, revealing healthier, brighter, and more radiant skin beneath. With properties to soothe sunburns, moisturize, hydrate, and calm sensitive skin, lactic acid is a multi-tasking powerhouse that gives milk its skin-perfecting abilities.

Besides, cow milk, goat milk and donkey milk all are lactose liquid rich with ceramides and hyaluronic acid. Have you ever tried milk skincare with donkey milk, goat milk, or even whole milk? Did it make a difference in your skin? If you've already tried cow's milk in your skincare routine, take it to the next level with donkey milk. Donkey milk has 60 times more Vitamin C than cow's milk, and it's full of fatty acids and ceramides (lipid molecules that form a protective layer on the skin to retain moisture) for intensely hydrated results. Put the milk to the test. Dip a cotton ball into whole milk and gently swab all over a clean face. Following the "oil dissolves oil" rule, the healthy fat in whole milk will help slough away any remaining oil-based impurities like sebum, sunscreen, and makeup, as well as exfoliate and lighten your skin. Rinse off with lukewarm water. If you have a bathtub, treat yourself to some "you time" and pour a few cups of milk into a tub of warm water.

The luxurious and silky mixture will leave your skin feeling ultra-soft and luminous. Not into playing with your food? Get the next best thing with milk protein-infused products like the Skinfood Milkshake Point Makeup Remover.

While milk may contain beneficial nutrients such as calcium and vitamin D, it's important to note that some people may be sensitive to milk or lactose intolerant. Additionally, over-cleansing or using harsh products can strip the skin of its natural oils and cause dryness or irritation. A gentle cleansing routine with a mild cleanser and moisturizer may be more appropriate for some individuals.

13.DAILY SKIN CARE FOR YOUTHFUL SKIN

Yes, skincare is vital. Your skin is the largest organ in your body, and it serves as a protective barrier against harmful environmental factors such as UV rays, pollution, and bacteria. Proper skincare can help keep your skin healthy and protect it from damage. Healthy skin looks better, feels better, and gives you more confidence. Skincare can help improve the texture, tone, and overall appearance of your skin. As you age, your skin naturally loses collagen and elastin, which can cause wrinkles, sagging, and other signs of ageing. Skincare can help slow down the ageing process and reduce the appearance of fine lines and wrinkles. Skincare can help prevent and treat acne by removing excess oil and dead skin cells, unclogging pores, and reducing inflammation. Taking care of your skin can be a form of self-care, helping you relax and feel better about yourself.

To keep youthful skin, demonologist suggests the minimum daily skin care would be morning cleaning and moisture and night cleaning and moisture. However, there are many mini-steps with toner, serum added for the routine. Here are these steps:

MORNING SKINCARE ROUTINE:

A morning skincare routine can help promote healthy, glowing skin throughout the day. Here are some steps you can take as part of a basic morning skincare routine:

(1) Cleanse: Start by cleansing your skin with a gentle cleanser to remove any oil or dirt accumulated.

(2) Tone: Use a toner to help balance your skin's pH levels and prep your skin for the next steps.

(3) Apply Serum: Apply a serum containing antioxidants, vitamin C, or hyaluronic acid to help protect and nourish your skin.

(4) Moisturize: Apply a moisturizer to help hydrate your skin and lock in moisture throughout the day. Choose a moisturizer that is appropriate for your skin type.

(5) Sunscreen: Apply sunscreen with at least SPF 30 to protect your skin from the sun's harmful UV rays. Apply a sunscreen that is appropriate for your skin type generously to all exposed skin.

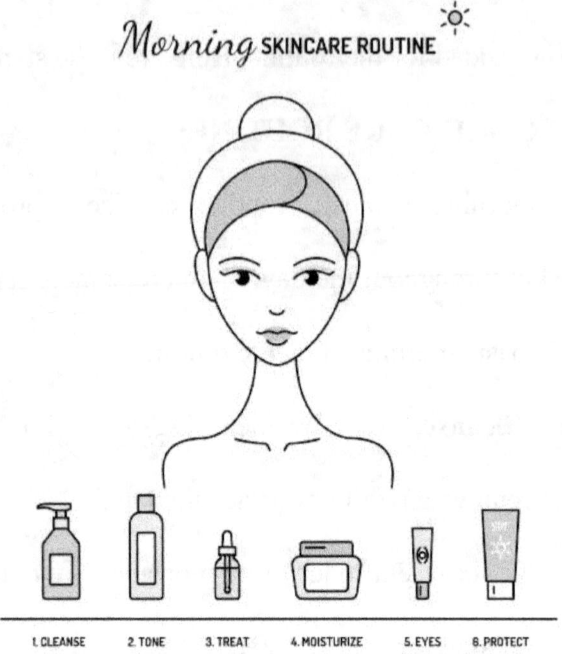

It's important to note that everyone's skin is different, and you may need to adjust your morning skincare routine based on your individual needs. For example, if you have oily skin, you may prefer a lightweight moisturizer or skip the moisturizer altogether. Conversely, if you have dry skin, you may want to use a more hydrating moisturizer or add a facial oil to your routine. In addition to a morning skincare routine, it's important to practice good overall skin care habits such as staying hydrated, getting enough sleep, managing stress, and avoiding smoking and excessive alcohol consumption.

NIGHT SKINCARE ROUTINE:

A night skincare routine can help promote skin repair and rejuvenation while you sleep. ***Here are some steps you can take as part of a basic night skincare routine:***

(1) **Cleanse:** Start by removing any makeup and cleansing your skin with a gentle cleanser to remove any oil, dirt, or pollutants that may have accumulated throughout the day.

(2) **Tone:** Use a toner to help balance your skin's pH levels and prepare your skin for the next steps.

(3) **Apply Treatment Products:** Apply any treatment products such as retinoids, acne medication, or skin-brightening agents.

(4) **Apply Eye Cream:** Apply an eye cream to the delicate skin around your eyes to help reduce the appearance of fine lines, wrinkles, and dark circles.

(5) **Moisturize:** Apply a moisturizer or facial oil to help hydrate your skin and lock in moisture overnight. Choose a moisturizer that is appropriate for your skin type.

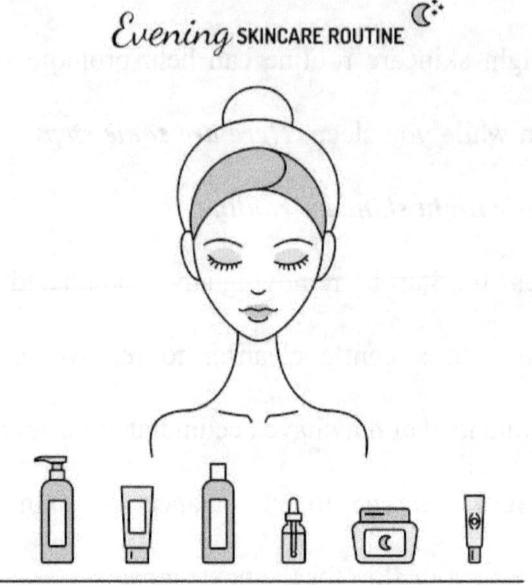

It's important to note that some treatment products, such as retinoids, can increase your skin's sensitivity to the sun. Be sure to apply sunscreen in the morning to protect your skin from UV damage. In addition to a night skincare routine, it's important to practice good overall skin care habits such as staying hydrated, getting enough sleep, managing stress, and avoiding smoking and excessive alcohol consumption.

14. KOREAN SKINCARE ROUTINE

Korean skincare routine is the very complicated and what most of us are obsessed with now. K-beauty care claims to provide perfect skin with a flawless and porcelain look. And it is true! Their 10-step skincare routine is an effective solution to achieving radiant and flawless skin.

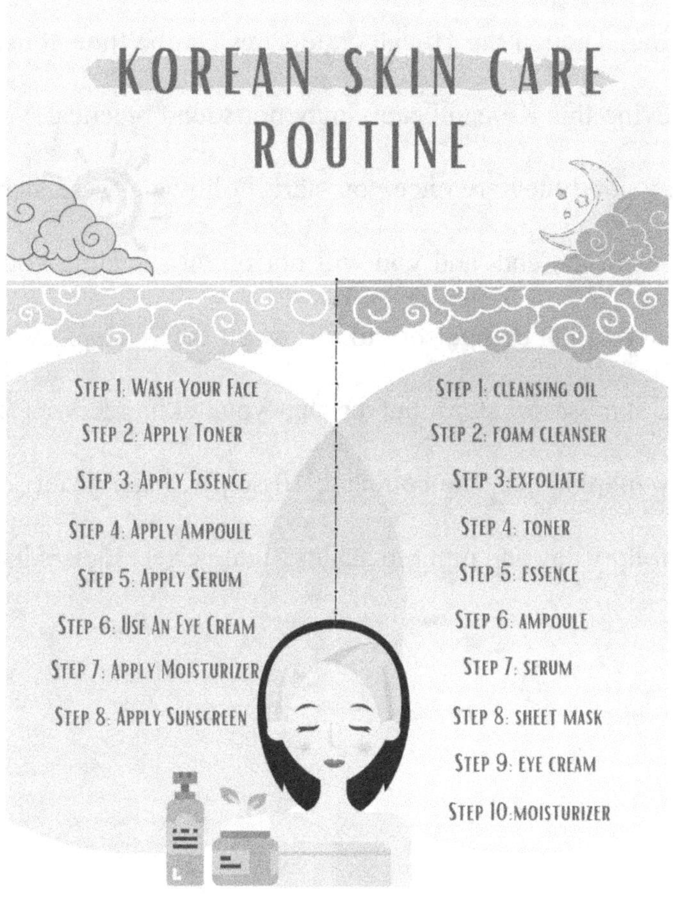

The Korean skincare routine is all about improving your skin health by moisturizing, keeping it hydrated, and offering the essential ingredients the right way. You can flaunt your natural skin without putting on any makeup. It involves using various hydrating products that assist in skin repair. This skin treatment prevents water loss and the entry of foreign substances through the skin. Furthermore, the processes help prevent fine lines, wrinkles, and other signs associated with ageing. Though the 10 elaborate steps can be time-consuming and achieving this Korean beauty may not sound practical, you will know how good they are once you start. Following these steps will be worth it in the end, and you will not regret spending your time doing this. It is not compulsory to follow all the 10 steps every day. You can skip some steps but ensure your skin receives all the necessary ingredients. The complete 10-step Korean beauty secrets you can follow day and night to achieve that perfect look is listed.

The 8-Step Korean Morning Care Routine!

- **Step 1:** Wash Your Face With Water

- **Step 2:** Toner

- **Step 3:** Essence

- ➢ **Step 4:** Ampoule

- ➢ **Step 5:** Serum

- ➢ **Step 6:** Eye Cream

- ➢ **Step 7:** Moisturizer

- ➢ **Step 8:** Sunscreen

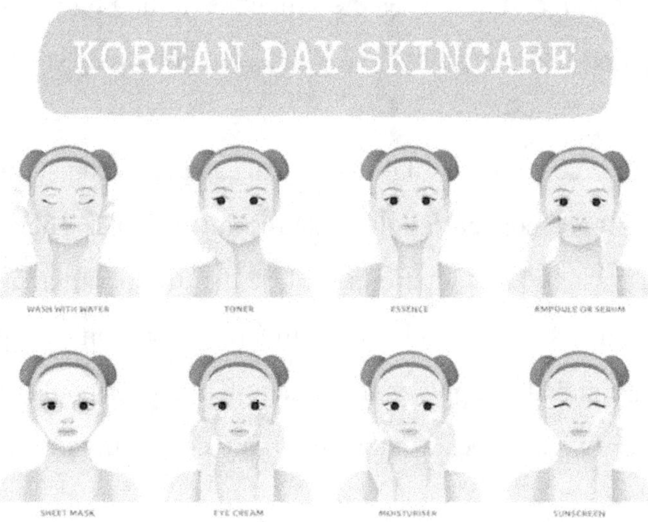

Step 1: Wash Your Face With Water

Use water to wash your face after you wake up. Do not use any cleanser. Water not only makes your skin feel refreshed, but it also removes impurities from your face that may have settled down on the skin during the night. It also keeps your skin hydrated.

Step 2: *Apply Toner*

After washing your face with water, apply toner. You may dab the toner on a cotton swab and apply it in a sweeping motion or pour the toner in your palms and pat it lightly all over your face. A toner helps to balance the pH level of your skin and ensures proper absorption of the next skincare products.

Step 3: *Apply Essence*

An essence is a blend of serum, toner, and moisturizer and is a crucial part of the 10-step Korean skin care regimen. It hydrates and primes your skin and nourishes the skin cells. Pour a bit of it on your palm and gently press it all over your face. Do not sweep your fingers.

Step 4: *Apply Ampoule*

Ampoules are similar to essences and serums, but they contain a higher concentration of active ingredients. They usually come in a glass bottle with droppers. Use the dropper to apply a few drops on your face. Use your fingers to tap and press it over gently. It is recommended to apply and massage Korean ampoules on your face once or twice a week as they are highly concentrated and active.

Step 5: *Apply Serum*

Serums are best for anti-ageing benefits and can reduce dark spots, hyperpigmentation, dryness, fine lines, and wrinkles. Take a pea-sized amount of serum (or two pumps) and press it gently all over your face with your fingertips.

Step 6: *Use An Eye Cream*

The area around your eyes is super delicate, you need an eye cream to keep the area hydrated and protected throughout the day. Take a little amount of eye cream on your fingertips and apply it from the inner corner of your eyes to the outer corners.

Step 7: *Apply Moisturizer*

Apply a layer of moisturizer on your face. A moisturizer keeps the skin hydrated, nourished, and radiant all day long. If you have oily skin, use a water-based moisturizer, and if you have dry skin, use a cream-based moisturizer. Massage the moisturizer gently all over your face and neck.

Step 8: *Apply Sunscreen*

Protecting your skin from UV rays is a must. Once you have completed all these steps, apply sunscreen. This prevents dark spots, tanning, sunburn, fine lines, and wrinkles. Use a product with at least SPF 30.

This is the elaborate 8-step Korean morning skincare routine. These products keep your skin hydrated and healthy throughout the day. A proper skincare routine makes sure that the skin heals and repairs itself properly.

The 10-Step Korean Night-time Routine!

- ➢ **Step 1:** Cleansing Oil
- ➢ **Step 2:** Foam Cleanser
- ➢ **Step 3:** Exfoliate
- ➢ **Step 4:** Toner

➢ **Step 5:** Essence

➢ **Step 6:** Ampoule

➢ **Step 7:** Serum

➢ **Step 8:** Sheet Mask

➢ **Step 9:** Eye Cream

➢ **Step 10:** Moisturizer

KOREAN NIGHT SKINCARE

oil cleaner	foam cleanser	exfoliant	toner	essence
serum	sheet mask	eye cream	moisturizer	SPF or night cream

Step 1: Clean Your Face With A Cleansing Oil

You have to take off the dirt, sebum, and impurities accumulated on your face. Using a cleansing oil binds the dirt with the oil and makes it easier for you to clean your skin thoroughly. Massage the oil thoroughly all over your face and neck. Wipe your face with a wet cotton wipe.

Step 2: Double Cleanse With A Gentle Foaming Cleanser

After oil-cleansing your face and removing all makeup and dirt, use a gentle foaming cleanser to clean your face. Pour some cleanser on your palm, add water, and rub your palms together to generate lather or foam. Apply it on your face and wash it off.

Step 3: Exfoliate Your Skin

This step should not be repeated more than two times a week. Exfoliation helps in scraping the dead skin cells and impurities from your face. This evens out your skin tone and promotes cell regeneration . You may use a chemical or enzyme-based exfoliant or a physical exfoliator (scrub) on your skin.

Step 4: Apply Toner

This step is similar to the step in the morning skincare routine. At night, your skin need a toner to maintain the pH levels.

Step 5: Apply Essence

The essence always follows the toner. Never miss this step as the essence is needed to keep your skin hydrated for the entire night.

Step 6: Apply Ampoule

Right after hydrating your face with the essence, apply an ampoule. The super ingredients and active agents in the product will help your skin regenerate and recharge itself throughout the night.

Step 7: Apply Serum

After you have applied the ampoule, apply the serum to the specific areas of concern. For instance, if it is an anti-acne serum, apply it to the affected areas. However, you can apply the serum all over your face and neck. This depends on whether you are using a serum for specific skincare issues or overall nourishment.

Step 8: *Apply Sheet Mask*

This is an absolute favourite of K-beauty followers. The sheet masks are saturated with a serum that contains essential active agents. These are suitable for all skin types. They provide deep hydration to your skin and also offer specific benefits, such as anti-ageing, anti-acne, hydration, and collagen-boosting effects, depending on your skin's requirements.

Step 9: *Use An Eye Cream*

Once your skin has absorbed all the goodness of the sheet mask, it is time to take care of your eye area. Apply an eye cream to keep the delicate skin around your eyes hydrated and nourished.

Step 10: *Apply Moisturizer*

Finish off with a night moisturizer. Applying moisturizer at the end seals all the ingredients and helps your skin soak up everything throughout the night. You will wake up with soft and supple skin.

The Korean skincare routine is popular across the globe for hydrating your skin and imparting a natural glow to your skin. The simple step of washing your face with water gets rid of the grime and prepares your skin for the next steps of the routine. Toners, essence, serum, eye cream, ampoule, and moisturizers, each play an equally important part in hydrating your skin, slowing down ageing, and preventing sunburns and acne. Even though the ten-step routine may

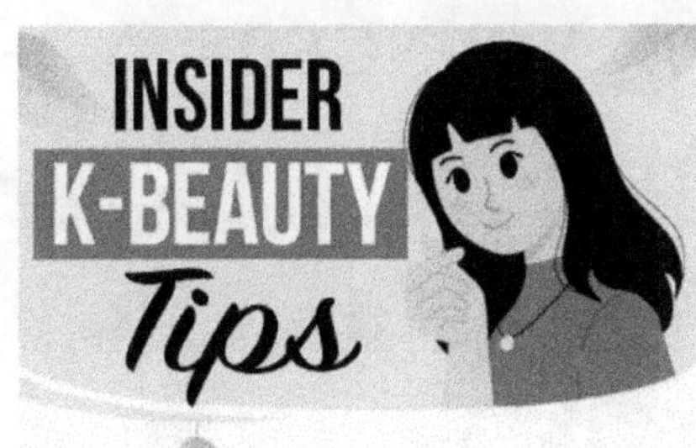

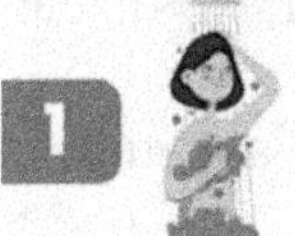

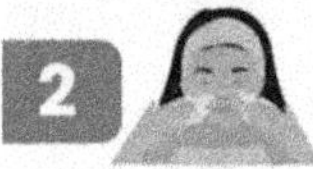

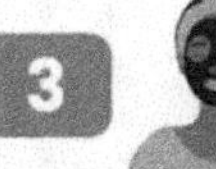
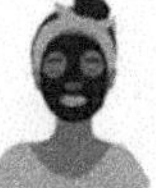

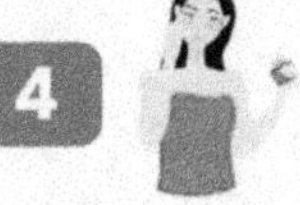

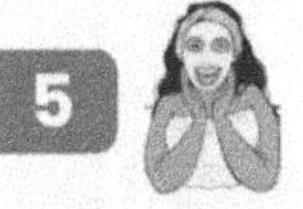

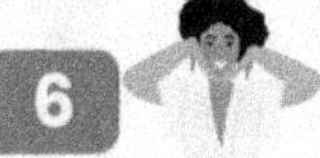

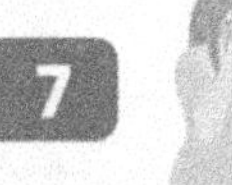
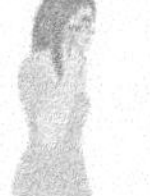

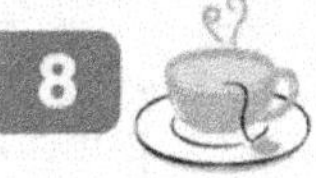

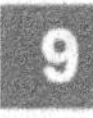

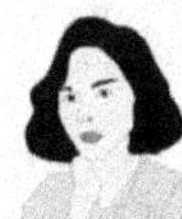
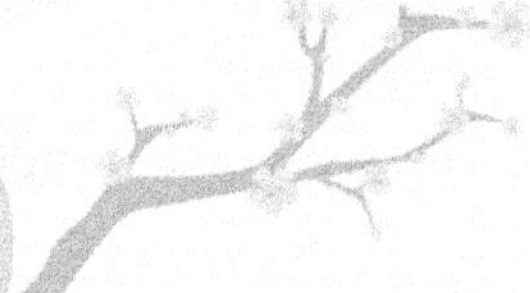

not seem practical at times, if you go through all the steps with patience and love, you will surely see the results over time. The Korean skincare routine is all about nourishing the skin and providing it with the right ingredients, both externally and internally. Here are a few additional tips that you may follow to keep your skin as healthy as the Koreans.

15. HOW TO LOOK YOUNGER

If you want to look younger right this second, there are plenty of ways to look more youthful and radiant. With just a few simple tweaks to your everyday skin care, makeup and hair routine, you can shave years off your appearance without having to spend a fortune.

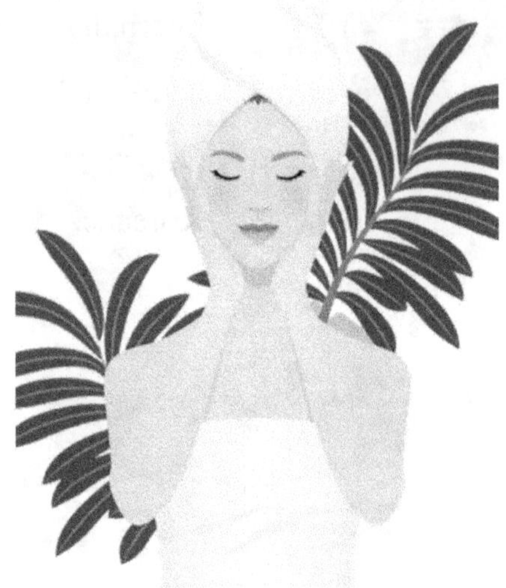

Here's what experts in skin care, hair care and cosmetics had to say about looking years younger, instantly.

(1) Use a Hydrating Mask: For tighter, glowing skin, put on a hydrating mask for ten minutes. The nourishing, hydrating ingredients plump your skin to make it appear more dewy and youthful with the appearance of fine lines reduced, such as Blue Marine Algae Intense Hydrating Mask

(2) Choose a Luminous Foundation: Not all foundations are created equal, and to best downplay those pesky fine lines and wrinkles, you'll want to choose a light-reflecting, lightweight, and luminous foundation. Steer clear of pressed powders or anything full coverage, as these products tend to settle into wrinkles. Instead, opt for a silicone-based, medium-coverage, liquid foundation or a tinted moisturizer with luminescent particles to easily create the illusion of a glowing complexion, such as Kevyn Aucoin – The Etherealist Skin Illuminating Foundation.

(3) Lighten Your Hair a Bit: A general universal rule is that the older you get, lighter colors will always look better. Not everyone looks good with blonde hair, but even traditionally dark-haired people can add a few highlights here and there. Not only do highlights help disguise grays, but they help prevent your hair from clashing with your complexion, as your skin tends to be less radiant as you age., such as Sun Bum – Blonde Hair Lightener

(4) Wear a Ponytail: If you're looking for a hairstyle that not only looks sophisticated but helps make your face look younger, you'll want to opt for a classic ponytail. When you pull your hair up into a ponytail—the higher the better—it helps raise the hair off of your face and gives you an instant mini facelift.

(5) Exfoliate (But Don't Overdo It): Making exfoliating part of your skin care routine can help brighten your skin on the spot. This takes away the dead skin and dullness that leads to looking older. Exfoliation helps to lessen the appearance of fine lines and wrinkles as well. Make sure to be gentle on your skin.

(6) White Out Your Waterline: You can avoid looking exhausted or dull by applying a little bit of light eyeliner to the inside of your eyes. Look bright-eyed and selfie-ready by using a gel liner (made for lining the inside rim of the eye). This will instantly create a well-rested, wide-eyed brilliance with a dash of youthful vivacity, such as Pixi by Petra – Eye Bright Liner

(7) Finish Your Look with a Mineral Mist: When all your makeup is done, use a mineral mist to add a beautiful glow to your skin in an instant. It will take away any makeup that became too dry and add glow instead. You can use this throughout the day to refresh the makeup.

16. COSMETIC TREATMENT OF SKIN

(1) USE A MOISTURIZER, THEN FOUNDATION

e.g. Hydrating Face Primer

As you age, your hormone levels drop and your skin gets drier.

While you may want to reach for a cream foundation, don't; because thicker, creamier formulas are usually made to provide fuller coverage, which means they're packed with more pigment. And pigment is basically powder. If you like a creamy formula's coverage, try it with a richer face moisturizer or a hydrating primer.

(2) TRY A COLLAGEN-BASED FACE CREAM

e.g. Elemis Pro-Collagen Marine Cream

We call collagen creams the "fountain of youth." If you like the sound of that, consider the Elemis Pro-Collagen Marine Cream, which is clinically proven to erase wrinkles. It's pretty pricey, but you should expect to see tightened, toned skin after 15 days.

(3) USE A CONCEALER FOR DARK CIRCLES

Estée Lauder Double Wear Stay-in-Place Flawless Wear Concealer

Keep under-eye concealer from drawing attention to your wrinkles, and apply it *only* on the inner halves of your under-eyes to cover up any darkness.

(4) KEEP YOUR EYE MAKEUP SIMPLE

Urban Decay Anti-Aging Eyeshadow Primer Potion

Oily lids could cause your eyeshadow to run, but that doesn't mean you should keep piling on product. Instead, apply a thin layer of a clear primer to hold everything in place. Then, apply flattering shadows like sage or jewel tones and use a liquid eyeliner to create that perfect line (without pulling and tugging on your skin).

(5) CURL THOSE LASHES--ULTA Eyelash Curler

Using an eyelash curler to open up your eyes. Lashes can make eyes look more youthful and awake. Take your curler and hold it for 15 seconds on each eye.

(6) APPLY SPF DAILY--Vichy LiftActiv Peptide-C Sunscreen SPF 30

Especially don't forget to apply a good sunscreen around your eye area. Eyelid skin (and the under eye area) is the thinnest in the body, so sun damage shows up quickly in this area in the form of dilating and increased blood flow. As a result, you can see a dark glow or color through the transparency of the skin.

(7) TAKE YOUR TIME REMOVING YOUR MAKEUP-- Clinique Take The Day Off Cleansing Balm

You might be excited to take off your makeup and hop in bed, but take your time with the removal process. That constant tugging and pulling at the delicate skin around the eye increases sagging and, as a result, can look darker than the skin around it. Consider using a cleansing oil or balm to remove mascara and eyeshadow with minimal tugging.

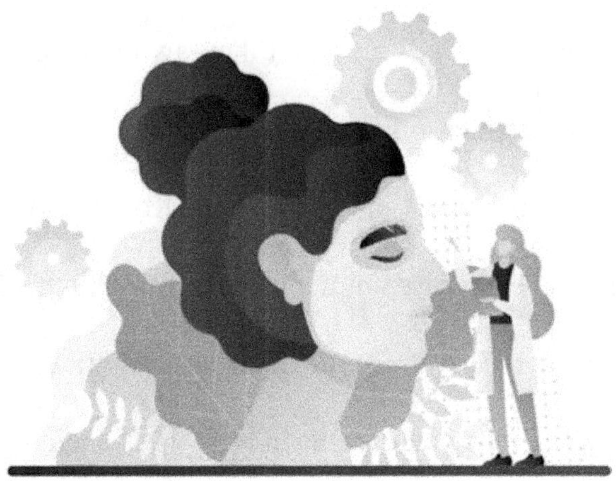

17. SIMPLE TREATMENT FOR YOUTHFUL SKIN

Overall, good skincare is important not only for your appearance but also for your health and well-being. By taking care of your skin, you can improve its health and appearance, and feel more confident and comfortable in your own skin! While milk, morning and night cleaning, and moisturizing can contribute to healthy skin, it's important to note that there are many factors that influence skin health and ageing. So it's important to take a holistic approach to skin health that includes a healthy diet, sun protection, hydration, sleep, and stress management. It's no secret that raw ingredients like milk, honey, fruits, vegetables, oils, and other natural products are used for their skin-enhancing perks in nearly every Korean skincare brand. Following are several easy, simple, yet effective skin treatments.

(1) **Apply milk to face every morning and night**: we have already gone through the components in milk that benefit our skin.

(2) **Egg white**: Apply egg white to skin as a mask can smooth the skin, and remove the wrinkles.

(3) Honey treatment: Apply honey to skin can tied up the skin and

remove wrinkles.

(4) Lemon and honey: can clean skin and remove acres.

(5) Butter: butter is a nature moisturizer,

(6) Coconut oil: coconut oil can whiten the skin;

(7) Aloe Vera: the juice from Aloe Vera can smooth the skin and

heal the scars.

(8) Steam as moisturizer: water fog or hot stream is a god moisture

for the skin too.

18. HEALTHY LIFESTYLE FOR

YOUTHFUL SKIN

Alongside diet, many external factors can shape our skin health, including our exposure to chemicals and sunlight, hydration levels and even how stressful our lives are. A healthy lifestyle includes a variety of habits and behaviours that promote overall health and well-being! A healthy lifestyle begin with a healthy diet or a balanced diet. A balanced diet that includes a variety of nutrient-dense foods, such as fruits, vegetables, whole grains, lean protein, and healthy fats, is essential for overall health.

Regular physical activity, such as cardio and strength training, can help improve cardiovascular health, strengthen muscles and bones, reduce stress, and improve mood.

Getting enough sleep is important for physical and mental health. It helps the body repair and rejuvenates itself, improves cognitive function, and supports a healthy immune system.

Chronic stress can have negative effects on physical and mental health. Finding healthy ways to manage stress, such as practising mindfulness, meditation, or yoga, can promote overall well-being. Avoiding harmful substances, such as tobacco, excessive alcohol, and drugs, can help prevent a variety of health problems.

Regular health checkups can help identify potential health problems early on and prevent them from becoming more serious.

By incorporating these habits into your daily life, you can help promote overall health and well-being. It's important to remember that a healthy lifestyle is a journey, and it takes time and effort to establish new habits and make lasting changes. *Here are some tips for a healthy lifestyle that can help promote healthy, glowing skin:*

1. **Stay Hydrated:** Keeping your body and skin hydrated is essential. Though topical ingredients will help your skin stay hydrated externally, you also need to provide internal hydration. Drinking plenty of water is important for maintaining healthy skin. It helps to keep your skin hydrated, which can improve its texture and appearance. Our skin needs to be hydrated to maintain a healthy level of elasticity. To achieve this, sip water throughout the day and aim to drink around 6 to 8 glasses of water. If your urine is darkly coloured, it likely means you are dehydrated.

2. **Follow a Balanced Diet:** A balanced diet that includes plenty of fruits, vegetables, whole grains, lean protein, and healthy fats can provide your skin with the nutrients it needs to look and feel healthy. Include fermented and pickled foods in your diet. Such foods contain essential vitamins and probiotics that are beneficial for both skin and gut health. Nourish your skin by eating a mix of colourful fruit and vegetables - at least 5 portions a day. Focus on getting more Omega 3's and

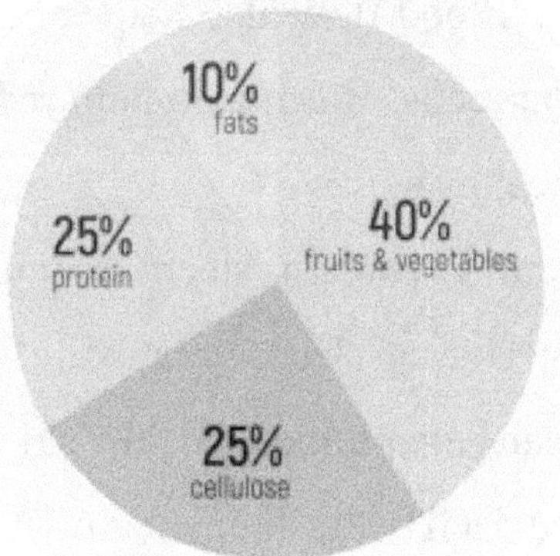

increase your skin's hydration from within. Flax, hemp and chia seeds and walnuts are great sources, as well as fatty fish such as herring, sardines, and salmon. Fish and meat broth contain collagen, which keeps your skin youthful and healthy. If you love having a dessert after meals, pick any fruit instead of baked and sugary delights. An effortless way is to blend a mix of veggies, fruit, and berries into a filling smoothie. And to try out new recipes to keep up a fun variety in your daily meals e.g., spinach and red pepper frittata, pumpkin pancakes, overnight carrot cake oats, or breakfast squash muffins.

3. **Exercise Regularly:** Regular exercise can help improve circulation, which can bring oxygen and nutrients to your skin. Getting the heart rate up will increase blood circulation, which in turn will deliver more oxygen and nutrients to the skin - thus boosting skin metabolism. Blood flow also helps remove toxins and free radicals from your cells. It can also help reduce stress, which can contribute to healthy skin.

4. **Get Enough Sleep:** Getting enough sleep is important for maintaining healthy skin. During sleep, your body repairs and rejuvenates itself, which can help promote healthy skin. When we sleep our bodies produce HGH, the human growth hormone, which kick-starts cell division that is essential to skin renewal and repair. During sleep our skin cells rebuild collagen and repair damage from UV exposure, fighting back wrinkles and age spots. Sleep deprivation has been shown to reduce skin elasticity and

gloss whilst aggravating wrinkles. Even one night of sleep deprivation can dehydrate our skin with visible results. Moreover, a lack of sleep can increase cortisol levels and potentially trigger acne and eczema breakouts.

5. **Manage Stress:** Chronic stress can contribute to a number of skin problems, including acne, wrinkles, psoriasis, eczema, and dullness. It has also been shown to have a detrimental effect on skin ageing. In short, stress prompts the adrenal glands to produce the stress hormone cortisol. In response, the sebaceous glands create more oil and sebum, which can clog the pores and result in acne breakouts. Additionally, stress can weaken the immune system and trigger inflammation, a condition known to aggravate psoriasis and eczema. Stress is also associated with dysbiosis in the gut and a number of complex diseases. Finding ways to manage stress, such as practising yoga or meditation, can help promote healthy, youthful-looking skin. Rest and relax, do not strain yourself. When you are stressed, it reflects on your skin. The best way to relax is by sleeping. When you sleep, your body restores and repairs itself. This improves your overall health (both physical and mental) and also benefits your skin. Take time to unplug & recharge, and focus on activities you genuinely enjoy, that bring peace to your mind and love in your heart.

6. **Minimize skin-damaging behaviour:** Don't drink alcohol or sugar calories. Avoid excessive sunlight, excessive sugar, and fatty foods for our skin to thrive.

7. **Don't smoke, and no drugs:** Smoking can accelerate the skin's ageing process by damaging collagen, producing free radicals in the body and narrowing blood vessels. All of these disrupt the ability of the skin to repair itself, making smokers look older than they are. Smoking can also exacerbate inflammatory skin diseases such as psoriasis due to its carcinogenic properties. Whichever way you cut it, quitting smoking is one of the best things you can do for skin health.

8. **Protect Your Skin from the Sun:** Ultraviolet light from the sun can damage your skin leading to wrinkles, dryness and even melanoma- the most deadly form of skin cancer. Exposure to the sun's UV rays can cause wrinkles, age spots, and other skin problems. Protect your skin by wearing sunscreen with an SPF of at least 30, wearing protective clothing, and avoiding the sun during peak hours. Never forget this even if it is cloudy and raining outside. UV rays can damage your skin and speed up the ageing process. Hence, carry your sunscreen along.

9. **Adapt your skincare to the seasons:** As the seasons change, so does the temperature, something which can influence your skin health significantly. In the winter months, cold weather can dry

out the skin resulting in flakiness, tightness and irritation. If you are already struggling with rosacea or eczema, cold weather can make these worse, as can the hot showers we often turn to in the winter months. A humidifier can counteract the effects of this and restore moisture to your skin, as can a gentle moisturiser. In the summer months, excessive sweating can lead to clogged pores and trigger acne breakouts. To prevent this, use a gentle non-alcoholic cleanser to wash your face after exercise, in the morning and before bed. A word of warning, though, excessive washing can strip the skin of its natural oils.

10. **Get enough vitamins:** Your skin thrives on a mix of vitamins, but most people do not get enough vitamins through their regular diet. Vitamin C is vital for the growth, development, and repair of all body tissues and is involved in many body functions, including the formation of collagen, absorption of iron, the proper functioning of the immune system, wound healing, and the maintenance of cartilage, bones, and teeth. Boost your Vitamin C intake and get more radiant and resilient skin in the process. Citrus fruits, papaya, kiwi, and broccoli are great sources of Vitamin C. Vitamin A is also essential to our skin and body health. Vitamin A helps protect the skin against UV damage, encourages the production of new skin cells, and stimulates collagen production, reducing wrinkles and slowing skin ageing. Vitamin A can be found in many healthy food options, but also in the form of retinoids in natural skincare products. Finally,

Vitamin E is also essential and has anti-inflammatory and skin healing properties, as well as reduces UV damage to the skin.

11. **Have a Consistent skincare routine:** A good skincare routine begins with a clean face. Pollution, dirt, sweat, and makeup should be removed so that the skin is ready for nourishing treatments and creams. Always thoroughly clean your face with a gentle cleansing product before going to bed, and in the mornings a quick rinse with water may be enough. Taking good care of your skin does not necessarily mean that you must have a complex routine. Be consistent and stick to something you are likely to repeat every day. The most important steps to implement daily are cleansing with a gentle cleanser, moisturizing with facial cream, and using an SPF30 sunscreen to protect the skin from external stressors. Once a week, it is also important to exfoliate your skin to remove dead skin cells and deeper impurities, and an adaptable exfoliating treatment is the best way to address your skin's changing needs. A good skincare routine also means paying attention to how your skin is feeling at a particular time of year or month and adapting your skincare products to suit this.

12. **USE GOOD QUALITY, NATURAL SKINCARE:** Skincare products can support your healthy lifestyle choices by providing an additional supply of nutrients and protection your skin needs to look and be healthy. But not all skincare products are created

equal! Always choose quality over quantity.Cheap skin care products are usually full of synthetic ingredients, mineral oil (petroleum) derivates, and cheap preservatives that do more harm than good in the long term. Instead look for all-natural skincare products that are formulated using only natural ingredients or nature-identical, clean molecules. Not only are natural beauty better for your skin health, but they are also much better for the environment.

A healthy lifestyle is very important for overall health and well-being. It can help reduce the risk of chronic diseases, such as heart disease, stroke, type 2 diabetes, and certain types of cancer. It also can improve energy levels and productivity, making it easier to perform daily tasks and activities. Regular exercise, a balanced diet, and stress management techniques can all help improve mood and reduce the risk of depression and anxiety. Maintaining a healthy weight through a balanced diet and regular exercise can help reduce the risk of obesity and related health problems. A healthy lifestyle can help prevent age-related declines in physical and cognitive function and support healthy ageing. By promoting overall health and well-being, a healthy lifestyle can enhance the quality of life and make it easier to enjoy daily activities and pursuits.

Overall, a healthy lifestyle is essential for physical and mental health and can help reduce the risk of a variety of health problems. By incorporating healthy habits into your daily routine, you can promote overall well-being and enjoy the many benefits of a healthy lifestyle! By following these tips and maintaining a healthy lifestyle, you can help promote healthy, youthful-looking skin that you'll be proud to show off!

19. HEALTHY RELATIONSHIP FOR YOUTHFUL SKIN

There's plenty of evidence out there that shows good relationships make us healthier in a variety of ways, but did you know they can also be good for your skin? Skin is our largest organ and there's a lot going on under the surface. Quite often, when something is amiss in your body it will show up in your skin. Likewise, your skin will also reflect good health. Interestingly, healthy relationships have been linked to good health and longevity – and your skin will reflect it. Here are three cool ways that a healthy relationship will make your skin glow. A healthy relationship can have a positive impact on both mental and physical health, which can in turn promote healthy skin. Here are some ways that a healthy relationship can benefit the skin:

(1)   **Reduced Stress:** stress can wreak havoc on our skin, making it dull, dry, and lifeless and contributing to acne. When you're stressed, your skin will often be one of the first areas in your body to start giving you clues. A healthy relationship can help

reduce stress levels, which can have a positive impact on the skin.

(2) **Emotional Support**: Emotional support from a partner can help improve mental health, wand also benefit the skin. Stress, anxiety, and depression all lead to skin problems; having a supportive partner can help reduce the risk of these issues.

(3) **Healthy Habits**: A partner who encourages and supports healthy habits, such as exercise, a balanced diet, and regular sleep patterns, can help promote overall health and well-being, which can benefit the skin.

(4) **Positive Attitude**: Being in a positive relationship can help improve mood and overall outlook on life, which can help reduce the risk of stress-related skin problems.

(5) **Risk of cardiovascular disease is lowered**: marital or relationship quality and loneliness play a significant role in heart health. When the heart is not healthy, the skin often has a greyish or bluish tint and appears dull. By contrast, the skin of a person with a healthy heart has colour in their cheeks and their overall skin has good colour and vibrancy.

(6)   **Get sick less and heal faster:** people in healthy relationships have stronger immune systems. They get sick less and heal faster. When you have a strong immune system, your body is better able to ward off illness and diseases which means a healthier you. Good health in and of itself will make your skin glow, but should you get a pimple it will heal faster.

Overall, a healthy relationship can provide emotional and physical benefits that can have a positive impact on the skin. By fostering a supportive and positive relationship, you can promote overall health and well-being, which can help keep your skin looking and feeling healthy. How Does being in a relationship affect your skin?

Social contact and supportive relationships are essential for good health and well-being. Being in love, especially, can impact your skin in ways you may not have thought about before! When relationships are brand new, you may be all over each other: hugging, kissing, and cuddling. These are all good things, as physical touch releases serotonin, the happy hormone, as well as oxytocin, which helps to ease stress and improve your mood. Oxytocin is a hormone associated with bonding, social behaviour, and attachment in mammals; it has been found to increase bonding-related behaviour, trust, and empathy (Schneiderman). These hormones also impact your skin by giving off a radiant, natural glow, which people tend to refer to as a "Love Glow."

As wonderful as the love glow is, incorporating your partner into your life may change your daily routine— your eating habits, sleeping habits, and hormone levels can all change for the better or worse. Changes in your exposome (sum of all environmental factors like daily routine, stress and nutrition) can have detrimental effects on your skin. Fun activities may include dining out or drinking more, which may also impact your sleeping patterns. Make sure to drink plenty of water as your drink since alcohol dehydrates the body, and try to stick to a diet full of healthy nutrients and meats, as fried, processed foods and sugar can cause the skin to become inflamed and not receive the nutrients it needs to look its best. Keep yourself accountable and plan activities, like a hike or run along the beach, for you and your partner to do together.

And with all the fun you're having, you may forget to take off your makeup or use a different skincare product. What's important is being consistent with your skincare routine. Keep a travel-size regimen with you to make sure your love glow doesn't interfere with your Lancer Glow.

Being in a relationship should be a beneficial experience—you better each other's lives by bringing out the best in each other—and that goes for your skin, too! Maintain your skincare routine as best as you can, and enjoy all the benefits a healthy, happy relationship can give you. Remember that routine and mental health affect your skin. Do what you can to keep yourself sane while enjoying your newfound love and don't forget that the most important relationship you will ever have is with yourself.

20. HAPPINESS THE MOST IMPORTANT SKIN CARE INGREDIENT

While negative emotions can contribute to skin damage, positive emotions help improve it. Happiness releases all the feel-good hormones like endorphins, serotonin, and oxytocin. These hormones help your body function properly, your blood circulates well, and oxygen is efficiently passed throughout your body. When you have well-distributed oxygen and nutrients it shows in your skin. You develop that happy glow. Additionally, you are avoiding the release of stress hormones that inhibit the production of helpful and healing collagen and elastin. Your skin is balanced and skin issues aren't as problematic. When you are happy, the symptoms are: clear, balanced, hydrated, plump, buoyant, and glowing skin. These aren't merely the markers of youthful skin but the appearance of your skin on happiness. Not only that but your skin's ability to repair and renew itself is enhanced. Overall, your skin looks healthy, radiant, and younger.

There's no denying the power of positive emotions in improving your skin. Sometimes called the "happiness glow", this theory believes that positive emotions can help repair and heal your skin, causing your skin to effortlessly look healthy and glowy.

Happiness is the most important skin care ingredient. The benefits go beyond just a lift in mood. Happiness reduces stress, which is responsible for a whole host of skin issues. Putting attention toward your happiness and emotional well-being can have a big impact on your outward appearance. Focus on things that bring you happiness and know that fleeting positivity isn't as helpful as lowering stress over time and learning to implement techniques to reduce the risk of health issues. Following the below ways to consistently bring happiness and joy into your life will make you feel loved and confident. Feeling loved, confident, and comfortable in your own skin will in turn make you happy and will naturally give you a more youthful, glowing appearance.

(2) Smiling:

One simple way to start is with a smile. Smiling rewires your brain toward greater happiness. Genuine smiles make for healthy, glowing skin. This is because smiling uses your brain's reward mechanism which ultimately stimulates endorphins and serotonin. These make you feel happy and over time improve your skin. It stimulates the brain's reward mechanism in much the same way that getting exercise does. Studies have shown that smiling provides a greater reward stimulus than eating 2000 bars of chocolate. Here's how it works. You watch a hilarious cat video or meet up with a great friend. Your neurons light up and send signals to the muscles in your face that create a smile. In turn, when you smile, your facial muscles send reinforcing messages back to the reward centre in your brain stimulating endorphins and serotonin. It's a feedback loop of joy. And it's making you instantly and infinitely more beautiful.

(3) Prioritizing Time With Loved Ones

Spend time with loved ones. This will surely put you in a positive attitude by being surrounded by those who love and appreciate you for being your unique self. By spending time building loving relationships instead of toxic relationships, you are setting yourself up for success in feeling genuine happiness instead of having to "fake a smile". Call your friends and/or family members weekly or spending time with them to put yourself in a good mood.

(4) Practice Relaxing Techniques To Reduce Stress

Another way to prioritize your happiness is by daily practising ways to reduce your stress levels. Stress is normal;

however, intense, chronic stress is harmful. Consider practising meditation, reading, doing yoga, or whatever method helps you manage your stress levels.

(4)Treat Yourself

Last but not least, it's important to treat yourself to make you feel the best, most confident version of yourself. At BB Aesthetic, we offer a wide range of services in a happy, comfortable space that will help improve your skin's youthful, dewy glow. From facials to chemical peels, you deserve to feel confident and happy to look and feel you are the very best.

Happiness is an essential component in having naturally glowing skin that lasts.

REFERENCES

1. https://www.goodhousekeeping.com/beauty/anti-aging/tips/g2154/125-ways-to-look-young-feel-great/

2. playfitness.com.au

3. science.org

4. National Library of Medicine

5. Exercise Right - Blog [Research Blog]

6. MedlinePlus (.gov)

7. Healthline.Com

8. Younger Skin Through Exercise - The New York Times

9. 5 face yoga exercises- India today

10. californiamobility.com Do Vegans Age Better? Experts Share Their Thoughts

11. livekindly.com The Reason a Plant-Based Diet Has So Many Anti-Aging ...

12. health.harvard.edu Becoming a vegetarian

13. beautytap.com Got Milk? Song Joong Ki's Secret for Brighter, Smoother Skin

14. Stylecraze - Korean Skincare Routine

15. LIFESTYLE HABITS FOR BEAUTIFUL SKIN - NUORI

16. Diet & Lifestyle Tips To Keep Your Skin Young and Healthy- atlasbiomed.com

17. lancerskincare.com

18. highereducationskincare.com

19. helloclue.com

20. drzenovia.com

21. thriva.com

22. ncbi.nlm.nih.gov

23. soonskincare.com

24. vivantskincare.com

25. bbaesthetic.com

ABOUT THE AUTHOR

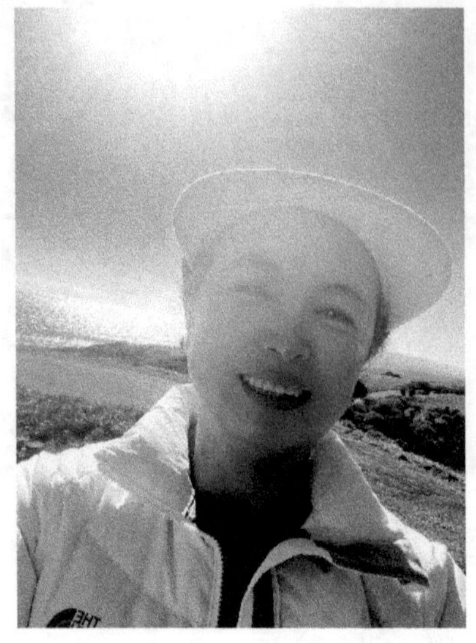

Susan Su holds a Ph.D. from U. C. Berkeley. She worked in the National Berkeley National Lab, consulted for National Aeronautics and Space Administration (NASA). She published many scientific papers at international and national journals. She is also a prolific author of fictions, non-fictions and screenplays.